Diabetes Management

The Ultimate Guide To Keeping Your Sugar Level In Control

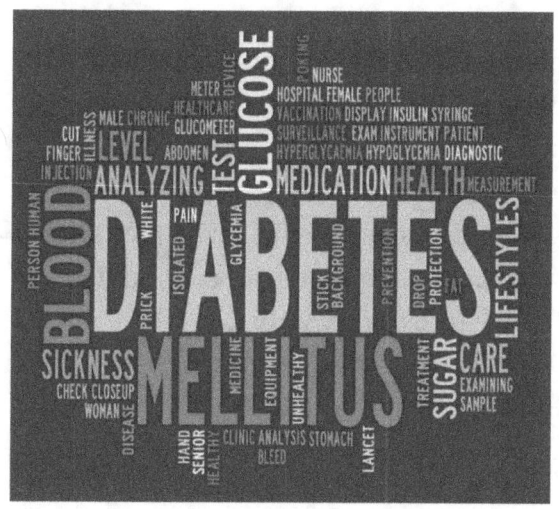

By

Fhilcar Faunillan

The trademarks that are used are without any consent, and the publication of the trademark is without permission or backing by the trademark owner. All trademarks and brands within this book are for clarifying purposes only and are the owned by the owners themselves, not affiliated with this document.

Table of Contents

INTRODUCTION

I want to thank you and congratulate you for downloading the book *"Diabetic Diet: The Ultimate Guide To Keeping Your Sugar Level In Control"*.

Diabetes is not new to all of us. We have probably heard of a friend, a family member or an officemate who has this real chronic disease. And the main reason why people acquire diabetes is because some people's sugar level is already beyond normal.

Way back when we were still kids, we really love to eat candies, chocolates, and all other foods that are sweet. This is because evolutionarily, people are inclined to liking sweet-tasting foods since it connotes that the food is safe and good to eat. However, the more we recognize that fact, the more we become addicted to it. But the problem does not stop there, in fact, that is where the bigger problem emerges. Most people who have high blood sugar level most often are not aware. Hence, this makes it a little harder for them to change their bad habits and lifestyle.

In Chapter 1, we will have a brief background about diabetes and a little of its biological implications.

In Chapter 2, all about types of diabetes and blood sugar level will be discussed. Read this chapter and discover some things about your blood sugar.

Of course, this book would not be complete if alternatives would not be discussed. So, for Chapter 3, we will talk about how to balance your plate—the type of food you should consume.

There are a lot of ways on how to control your blood sugar level. Every individual is unique, thus everyone also has different methods in facing this problem. But in this book, for sure you will be able to find one or all of the methods effective. Some of them may work and some of them may not be as effective as the other methods, but it would be to your benefit to try them all out and see which one or a combination of them is most effective in your lifestyle.

Now, what are these ways? Will it be easy? I tell you, it will never be easy, but it is very possible.

In this book, you will learn a lot of essential information about diabetes, blood sugar level, and how to keep your sugar level in control.

This book aims to inspire, give hope and inform people that it is never too late to make a big shift of your ways of living. We will take matters into our own hands and take the necessary steps to taking care of our health. There will be tips on having the proper mindset, dietary planning, and especially, lifestyle changes.

Again, I want to thank you and congratulate you for downloading this book. I hope this will be the beginning of your lifestyle change. Enjoy reading and learning!

Chapter 1- What You Should Know About Diabetes

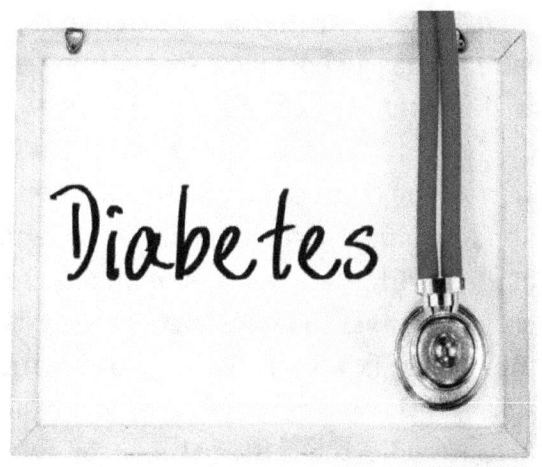

Diabetes is a common term we hear of nowadays. Worldwide, or even around us, a lot of people have been faced with this dreaded disease. But, did it even come to our minds what diabetes really is? Have we questioned why it does affect almost everyone? And have you ever wondered why it is one of the most leading causes of death?

Diabetes, as used repeatedly through time, is the shortened term for the real chronic ailment called scientifically as diabetes mellitus which is characterized by an increase in the body's sugar level. Diabetes has been taken from the Greek word *siphon* which means the flow of liquid from higher to lower level. Taking back to the 2nd century A.D., Arêtes the Cappadocian, a Greek physician likened patients with diabetes to siphons as they pass too much water. *Mellitus* on the other hand is also a Greek word which refers to the flow of sweet blood inside our body and the outward flow of sweet urine. In addition to that, *Mel* in Latin means "honey". Take note that diabetics' blood and urine contain high glucose level, which is then described to be as sweet as honey. From the etymology presented, diabetes mellitus then means the "siphoning of sweet water" or the "flow of sweet water".

Our body has its own ways of protecting us from different diseases. However, when one has diabetes, he or she loses the power and natural ability to convert glucose into energy. This happens due to many reasons: first, it could be that, most often the insulin production is inadequate and sometimes the cells in our body do not respond properly to insulin. Insulin is a hormone that gives support to our cells so that they can utilize glucose for our energy conversion. People with high blood sugar will typically experience polyuria or frequent urination, which then results to polydipsia (extreme thirst) and polyphagia (extreme hunger).

Chapter 2- Types of Diabetes

TYPES OF DIABETES

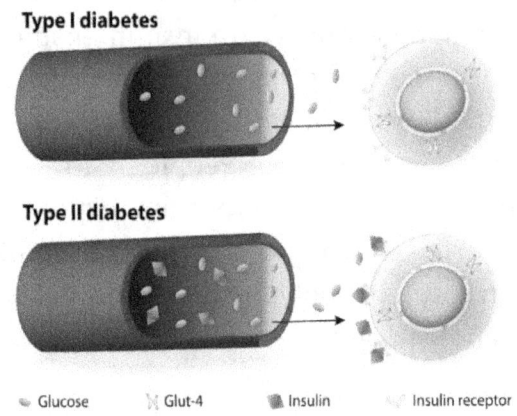

Type I diabetes

Type II diabetes

Glucose   Glut-4   Insulin   Insulin receptor

Diabetes is of various types, some of which are more dominant than others. There are however three main types of diabetes.

1. **Type 1 diabetes.** Also referred to as juvenile, early on-set, or insulin-dependent diabetes, Type 1 diabetes is an autoimmune condition by which the pancreas fails or produces insufficient

amount of insulin, a hormone responsible in allowing glucose to penetrate the cells to produce energy. As the name implies, this type of diabetes occurs among children and adolescents but is not limited to this age group as it can also manifest among adults. However, we should not put all the blame to our genetic compositions and family history. Geography and culture are also part of the risk factors for this disease. According to studies, the incidence of type 1 diabetes tends to get higher as you travel away from the equator. In addition to that, some studies suggest that people residing in Finland and Sardinia have the highest incidence of type 1 diabetes — about two to three times higher than rates in the United States and 400 times the incidence among people living in Venezuela. Type 1 diabetes is only found in five to ten percent of patients and occurs during childhood or in mature people that is why this is nowhere near as common as Type 2 diabetes.

The signs and symptoms of Type 1 diabetes patients include extreme hunger and thirst, unexpected weight loss, frequent urination, blurred vision, mood swings and increased irritability, extreme fatigue and weakness, bedwetting among children who have no previous bedwetting history, and vaginal yeast infection among women. This can affect major organs in your body, including the heart, blood vessels, nerves, eyes. If let alone, this can lead to blindness and kidney failure. Not only does genetics cause this occurrence but viruses as well. Should you notice any of these conditions, see your doctor right away. While there is no cure for this condition, its effects can be minimized with proper treatment and controlled food blood glucose levels and overall lifestyle change. Many patients with this type of condition have lived healthy and normal lives with constant discipline.

Keeping your blood sugar level close to normal most of the time can dramatically and gradually reduce the risk of many complications. Unfortunately, patients with this type of diabetes need to take injections for the rest of their lives and must monitor their blood glucose levels by undergoing regular blood tests by strictly following a special and healthy diet prepared by their physician or a registered nutritionist.

2. **Type 2 diabetes**. This is the most common disease throughout the world. More than 90% of those

diagnosed with diabetes fall under this classification. According to clinical studies, in America alone, there are 25 million people diagnosed with diabetes. Can you imagine how many people have this kind of disease throughout the world? In this kind of diabetes, our body generally produces insulin; however, it could be that the amount of insulin is not enough to support our body, or sometimes our body cells become resistant to it, compared to the first type of diabetes in which the body does not produce insulin at all.

There are some though who have been lucky enough to control and regulate the symptoms by decreasing their weight, maintaining a healthy and well-balanced diet, performing various exercises in moderation and closely monitoring blood glucose levels. Despite these, there are instances where this type of diabetes may progress and get worse thereby causing patients to take in insulin tablets.

The risk of developing Type 2 diabetes is higher among overweight and obese individuals (especially those with belly fat or suffering from central obesity) than those with a normal body weight. Why is that so? The reason is that, excessive body weight induces the body to discharge chemicals that would destabilize its metabolic and cardiovascular systems. If you have been inactive all your life, have a stagnant routine or what is termed as a couch potato, you are potentially at risk of having this disease.

Here's more. The love for soda has been undeniably contagious. Since the day you began to love these thirst quenchers, you embrace the risk of having this type of diabetes by 22%. Sugary drinks such as sodas have a direct impact on diabetes risk rather than weight gain.

Age likewise plays a huge role in Type 2 diabetes. This is prevalent among individuals falling under the age of 25-75. As you get older, the risk of having the disease become higher as physical activities becomes lesser compared to youngsters.

Gender is another factor. Various studies have shown that men with lower levels of testosterone are more at risk as this has been associated with insulin resistance.

3. **Gestational Diabetes.** Most people have the slightest idea what this type of diabetes is. Gestational diabetes greatly affects women during their pregnancy period.

There are women with extremely high blood sugar levels and their overall body process is incapable of producing the amount of insulin necessary to distribute glucose into their cells which results to progressive rising glucose levels. Majority of the patients with gestational diabetes were able to regulate their condition with proper exercise and balanced diet. Unlike the other types of diabetes, the percentages of patients who take in blood glucose control medications are only between 10-20%. However, there are patients who are not able to control their diabetes, which results to complications of sorts during childbirth and their babies will have to suffer the consequences of having gestational diabetes mellitus. Their new-born babies are larger than he or she should normally be. Also, it has been found that mothers whose diets were concentrated with animal fats, oil and cholesterol before they were impregnated have a higher risk for gestational diabetes, compared to those who have them in lesser amounts. Animal fats and oils are naturally-occurring molecules derived from different domestic animals like pigs, cows, and chickens.

Diabetes is a very high maintenance and sensitive illness wherein you need to monitor and regulate your blood sugar levels constantly. What is worse, diabetes is a chronic disease which means that once you have it, you will have it for the rest of your life.

Chapter 3 - Blood Sugar Level And Its Significance

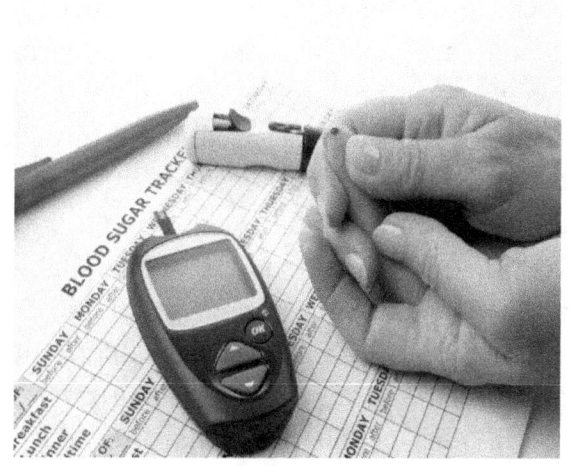

What really is blood sugar? How do we acquire a high blood sugar level? And what happens when it is too high?

Glucose, or what is commonly known as the blood sugar concentration, is the amount of sugar found in your blood and body. It mainly comes from the food you eat, and it is your body's main source of energy. Your blood transports glucose to all of your body's cells to use for energy.

People acquire a high blood sugar level through one major reason, and that is sugar addiction. Just like any other addiction, it is most difficult to stop because in the evolutionary perspective, people are naturally inclined to eating sweet tasting foods. And almost everywhere, there is an abundance of it, thus makes people lose control and indulge. Unfortunately, no rehabilitation facilities for sugar addicts are available; and worst part is that most people do not even recognize it as a real problem and often refer to it as simply having a sweet tooth. Most people find it hard to believe that sugar is addictive. It is because we associate addiction with sex, alcohol, smoking, drugs, and other things which are considered taboo by a society and sugar is not taboo. But in reality, many people suffer from it without being aware of it. Sugar addiction or overdependence on all foods containing any form of sugar leads to a lot of diseases, with obesity being one of the most common and diabetes, one of the leading causes of mortality in the world.

It was mentioned above that people are naturally inclined to liking sweet foods, so what makes it bad for our health? During the olden times, our ancestors depend on natural sweeteners. By natural, it means that they got it from fruits, plants, and vegetables, which is contrary to what we have now. Most of us depend on processed foods which satisfy the same cravings we had with our ancestors, but we get ours from a different and unnatural sources.

Now, the question is what happens to our body when our blood sugar level is too high? What are its effects? The effects could be is that we may acquire diabetes. And second, it could lead to obesity. We now have what the medical world calls as the "obesity epidemic". This does not mean that when you go around hanging out with obese people, you also become obese. But this means that most of the population right now are obese or overweight, with the food industry being what it is, the challenge just grew to greater heights. And obesity comes with it a range of deadly diseases like high cholesterol, hypertension, stroke, and heart disease.

Hyperglycemia is the scientific term for having a high blood sugar level. When this happens, the most common symptoms would be having a dry mouth, being thirsty most of the time, frequent urination, blurred vision, and over time, weight loss without even trying.

When your blood sugar stays too high for a long time, it can damage blood vessels and nerves. This damage can affect many of the organ systems in your body and can raise your risk of complications of stroke, heart diseases, eye problems, dental problems, kidney diseases, or even sexual dysfunctions.

Nobody wants to talk about the bad effects of having a high blood sugar level, but let's face it. However, the good news is that that you can help avoid these problems by controlling your diabetes and taking good care of yourself. This means taking steps to lower your blood sugar levels.

Chapter 4 - Start Slowly

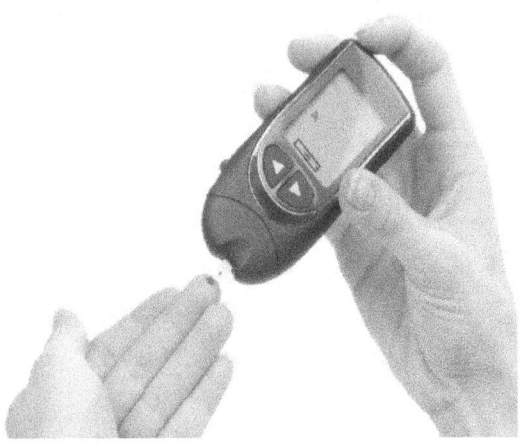

You have come across of the common adage, *"slowly but surely"*. True enough. In everything we do, especially in lifestyle changes, we must always start slowly.

1. Before you make changes, it is important to know and understand what you are dealing. The blood sugar concentration is the amount of glucose present in one's body. If the blood sugar level is too high, the body usually suppresses appetite over the short

term. Thus, **start by checking your blood sugar.**

How do you check your blood sugar level?

- First, you need to wash your hands with soap and clean, running water.
- After washing your hands, insert a test strip into your meter.
- Next, use your device on the side of your fingertip to get a drop of blood.
- Now, touch and hold the edge of the test strip to the drop of blood, and wait for the result.
- Lastly, your blood glucose level will appear on the meter's display.

Just in case you find it difficult to check your own blood sugar level, you may ask for help from a physician.

What does the result mean?

When you are done with the blood glucose check, keep a record of your results. Next, review them to see how your food intake, daily routine and activities and stress affect your blood glucose level. Now, take a closer look at your blood glucose record to see if your level is too high or too low for several days in a row at about the same time. If the same thing keeps on happening, you might want to consider changing your lifestyle. Work with your doctor or diabetes educator to learn what your results mean for you. Of course, this takes time, but please be patient enough. Ask your doctor or nurse if you should report results out of a certain range at once by phone.

Always put in mind that blood glucose results often trigger strong feelings and emotions. Blood glucose numbers can leave you confused, disappointed, upset, frustrated, angry, or down. It is so easy to use the numbers to judge you. Remind yourself that your blood glucose level is a way to track how well your diabetes care plan is working. It is not a judgment of you as a person. The results may show you the need for a change in your diabetes plan.

2. Setting your goals is pretty easy; however, achieving them is not. That is why, as much as possible, you have to keep your goals **SMART.**SMART goal setting provides structure and easier tracking of your goal including other things you want to achieve. Instead of formulating vague and general resolutions, SMART goal setting creates verifiable trajectories towards a certain objective, with clear milestones and an estimation of the goal's attainability. Every goal or objective, from intermediary step to overarching objective, can be

made S.M.A.R.T. and as such, brought closer to reality.

Now, what are these SMART goals? SMART goals stand for *Specific, Measurable, Attainable, Realistic and Time-bound* goals.

- **Specific.** It is important to make your goal focused and very well-defined. Most people find it easy to make general goals; yet, a specific goal has a much greater chance of being accomplished compared to that of a general goal. So how do you set a specific goal? You must be able to answer the six common and simple "W" questions: Who? What do I want to achieve, the conditions and the limitations? Where? When? Which? And why exactly do I want to reach this goal?

- **Measurable.** In order to be successful in achieving your goal, it should be measurable.

Measurable goals means there is a need for you to identify exactly and accurately what it is that you will see, hear and feel in the future when you reach your goal. It means breaking your goal down into measurable elements. You will need concrete and tangible evidence. Being happier is not evidence since this is subjective; not smoking anymore because you adhere to a healthy lifestyle where you eat vegetables twice a day and fat only once a week, is. Measurable goals can go a long way in refining what exactly it is that you want, too. Defining the physical manifestations of your goal or objective makes it clearer, thus easier for you to reach and achieve. You need to establish concrete criteria for measuring progress toward the attainment of each goal you set. It is important to measure your progress because it helps you to stay on track, reach the target dates you have set, and experience the euphoria achievement that spurs you on to continued effort required to reach your goal. Now, to determine whether your goal is measurable or not, you must be able to answer the questions, "How much? How many? How will I be able to maintain it if I have already reached my goal?"

- **Attainable.** Are your goals attainable? You have to investigate whether the goal really is acceptable to you. You weigh the effort, time and other costs your goal would take against the gains and the other obligations and the priorities you have in life. By the time you are able to identify your goals, you start to figure out the possible ways you can turn them into reality. You should develop the right attitude, skills, and abilities in order to reach them. Your goals become doable when you plot your steps carefully and create a schedule that allows you to carry out those steps. When you lost your goals, you are a step closer to them because it allows you to match them with the qualities you possess. Thus, making your goals within your reach, not because they are too easy to achieve, but because you have built yourself to combat them.

- **Realistic.** The common mistake people commit when they set their goals is that they become too idealistic. Let us face the truth, not everything is achievable. Therefore, we need to be realistic. To be realistic means you have to acknowledge your strengths and weaknesses, the possible and the things you are able to do.

- **Time-bound.** A goal should be grounded within a time- frame. Goals should be linked to a timeframe that creates a practical sense of urgency – that kind of putting up a schedule which results in tension between the current reality and the vision of your goal. Without such tension and motivation, it is unlikely for the goal to produce a relevant outcome.

Chapter 5 - Balance Your Plate

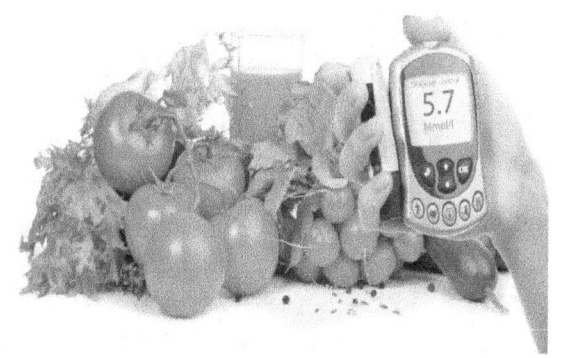

Closely monitoring your blood sugar levels and keeping its balance, a very strict and tight implementation of your diabetes diet plan, exercising regularly yet avoiding stress, and other lifestyle changes are crucial to avoiding the possible complications associated with the disease and maintaining energy levels.

You should note that you should be mindful with whatever you put into your mouths. The type of food you consume highly impacts your blood sugar level.

Thus, be sure to have the right kind and amount of food. Always practice healthy eating habits. Learn to balance your plate. If you are wondering how, here are some of the many ways available:

1. **You have to be smart in choosing your bread.** Bread is a part of our daily routine—from breakfast up until late midnight snacks. That is why, it is important to choose bread that is rich in fiber and protein because aside from the fact that it keeps your stomach feeling full and satisfied, fiber and protein slow down the absorption of glucose and decrease possible insulin rises.

2. **Drink moderately.** Drinking alcoholic beverages is not really bad at all because once in a while, our body needs it, as long as you do it moderation. Perhaps you have heard of the benefits of red wine to the cardiovascular system. Studies suggest that drinking a

glass of wine or a can of beer after dinner cut people's risk of having diabetes to about fifty percent compared to teetotalers since drinking the beverages result in a sudden drop in the insulin in the person's blood. As glucose does not easily get in, there is a huge tendency of artery damage.

3. **Consider dairy.** Drink at least two servings of low-fat dairy products a day. According to studies, it turns out that the lactose, protein and fat in dairy products improve blood sugar by filling you up and slowing the conversion of food sugars to blood sugar.

4. **Begin your day with a grapefruit.** Do not forget to include grapefruit in your breakfast tomorrow. Researchers found that patients who consumed grapefruit were able to shred about 3.6 lbs. off their weight. Not

only that. They each meal consisting of grapefruit resulted in having lower levels of glucose and insulin thereby increasing sugar metabolism as a result.

5. **Eat regularly.** Contrary to what is commonly done by other people, never ever skip meals, especially breakfast. Whenever you starve yourself, your blood sugar drops drastically causing shakiness and headache. The moment you put in something into your mouth, you get an overload of glucose and the pancreas is then pressured to release more insulin. This forced cycle is not at all recommended. Have a hearty and full breakfast then have smaller meals throughout the day. Most doctors advise eating every three to four hours to keep your blood sugar level normal and to control irregular eating behaviors. Do not wait until you are starving to eat,

instead eat when you are feeling only slightly hungry so you would have enough brain power to make healthier choices and eat in smaller amounts. So, start slow and start with making healthier choices for your food.

6. **Go nuts**. Literally, go nuts over nuts. When you make your salad, sprinkle a few slivered walnuts over it. Walnuts are great sources of monounsaturated fat, which won't raise your blood sugar as many other foods do. And some researchers suspect that this fat even makes cells more sensitive to insulin, helping to combat high blood sugar.

7. **Why not try buckwheat?** Eat the Japanese pasta which is made from buckwheat, a grain that helps in lowering blood glucose levels and it is rich in fiber, too!

8. **Make spinach your best friend.** Never forget to include spinach salad during dinner as your side dish. Spinach is high in magnesium, which a large study suggests can help to prevent the development of type 2 diabetes. Well, you can even have it with your favorite smoothie as a healthy refreshment.

9. **Watch your fat intake.** Reduce and cut back on saturated fat because those bloods with the highest levels of saturated fats were twice as likely have a high blood sugar level which leads to developing diabetes.

10. **Decaf.** It cannot be avoided that you would be tempted to eat that cake your partner baked, so you better pair it with a cup of decaffeinated coffee. While consumption of pastries like cakes, cookies and doughnuts can cause a

rise in the blood sugar level, pairing it with decaf coffee hampers blood sugar level from rising. You won't have the same effect if you would consume regular coffee. Do you know why? Though sugar absorption through your intestines is slowed down, caffeine also prolongs the reaching of sugar in the muscles. With that, sugar stays longer in the bloodstream.

11. **Go crazy over legumes**. These high-fiber foods take longer to digest so they release their glucose more slowly. According to studies, just consuming legumes of about 75 grams a day can help to stabilize blood sugar and insulin levels.

12. **Drink more and more water.** Water keeps your brain oxygenated which strengthens your willpower and curbs all your

eating impulses. This is also one of the perfect ways to keep your cravings from going out of control because you just might be dehydrated. In addition to that, water keeps your brain oxygenated which then again helps in strengthening your willpower and curbing all your eating impulses. Moreover, water is a good detoxifying agent to flush out all the glucose and toxins in your intestines. Moreover, water cleans up your palate and the taste buds of your tongue, which hastens the desensitization for sweet tasting foods. And lastly, water is a good detoxifying agent to flush out all the glucose and toxins in your intestines.

13. **Choose oatmeal over other carbs.** Oatmeal contains carbohydrate; however, it is a very good source of carbohydrate. Oatmeal can help control blood

sugar level. It is high in soluble fiber, thus, it is slower to digest and it won't raise your blood sugar as much or as quickly. It's going to work better at controlling blood sugar over time.

14. **Plan your meals.** It would be easy for you to avoid super sweet and unhealthy foods if you have planned your meals a day or week ahead. When you go to the grocery store, make it sure that you have listed everything that you needed.

15. **Know the difference between being bored and being hungry.** There are times when we confuse boredom with hunger. Have you ever noticed that when you have nothing to do, you find yourself going to the kitchen and looking for something to eat? Thus, this confusion leads to unhealthy eating patterns. A lot of people are guilty of using hunger as an excuse

to eat boredom. To make things clearer, there are times when our brain creates the same manifestation for both hunger and boredom. However, the difference is that when you are bored, your body just wants to do something compared to being hungry where anything will quell and suffice the grumbling stomach. Hence, take note of your eating schedule and compare that time for when you're feeling hungry. If it's out of schedule then you are more likely just bored.

16. **Go for the natural way.** Never ever think of replacing sugar with artificial sweeteners, because they don't work. The artificial sweeteners that you often find in "sugar-free" food and beverages will do nothing but increase your craving and wanting for sugar. The goal here is to stop wanting sugar and not just losing weight. Hence,

if you continue to trick your brain into liking sugar, then you will never lose your sugar cravings.

17. **Consume foods that are rich in fiber.** While there are dietary fibers that do not supply calories or nutrients, they positively affect your blood sugar level. Soluble fiber, which is water soluble, can stabilize blood sugar levels as it helps in postponing stomach emptying. With that, carbohydrate absorption is slowed down causing the blood sugar regulation to improve and the body's insulin requirements are lowered. Insoluble fiber on the other hand, which is non-liquid soluble including water, helps in increasing waste elimination, thereby preventing constipation. When planning for your meals, consider including leafy vegetables, spinach, broccoli, green beans, and kale as these

contain no starch and have lower carb content. Other fibrous sources though rich in starch include beans, potatoes, fruits, lentils, corn, pasta, cereals, peas, whole-grain breads and winter squash.

18. **Eat foods that are rich in antioxidants.** You surely have heard of free radicals. These are molecules containing unpaired electrons that can cause potential damage to the cells and even diseases. Antioxidants then work as a natural defense against these free radicals. What is its significance to diabetes?

19. **Consume antioxidant-containing foods.** Patients with diabetes have very low levels of antioxidants and increased levels of free radicals. For that reason, increased intake of sources of antioxidants from zinc, vitamin E

and selenium is encouraged. Among the best sources antioxidants are tomatoes, bell peppers, squash, cherries and blueberries. Walnuts and seafood are rich in selenium while whole grains, wheat germ and leafy greens are rich in vitamin E. Zinc can be obtained from seafood sources, nuts, red meat, poultry, beans, and fortified cereals.

20. **Consider including healthy fats.**
Not all fats are unhealthy. Including these along with carbohydrates in your diet is recommended. Excessive consumption of processed foods which are relatively easier to digest can cause a significant rise in one's blood sugar level thereby making one prone to Type 2 diabetes and insulin resistance. The inclusion of healthy fats from fish, canola and olive oil in your diet can slow down the digestive

process and buffer carb absorption. Note however that you should shun yourself from consuming saturated fats found in processed and fried foods.

21. **Focus on what you are eating.** With the different gadgets we have nowadays, not to mention our access on the internet, people find it hard to focus on what they are doing, especially eating. And this sometimes leads to multitasking. But getting distracted while eating might lead to overeating or eating the wrong foods, and worse, you are unaware of it! Studies have shown that we actually eat more when we do not notice that we are eating.

22. **Try out some smoothies.** This is probably the newest trend right now. A lot of people go crazy about smoothies. They do not only help you in losing weight; moreover, it

helps you control your blood sugar level, only if they are made from natural ingredients, and not from artificial sweeteners.

23. **Spice it up.** You may want to try cinnamon. It helps in reducing blood sugar and reducing the risk for developing type 2 diabetes. A clinical study revealed that both whole cinnamon and extracts has the effect of lowering fasting blood glucose. Also, there is a kind of spice called *fenugreek*. Similar with the cinnamon, this also reduces blood sugar level in people with both type 1 and type 2 diabetes as well as those with pre-diabetes. Fenugreek is also full of vitamins, minerals, and antioxidants. It can be taken as a pill, but it can also be consumed as a tea, or added to a wide variety of tasty recipes.

24. **Eat your colors.** Blueberries and red cherries are awesome source

of soluble fiber and it contains a number of other important nutrients and antioxidants. According to a study conducted last 2010 there are benefits of adding blueberries to the diet of obese people who had pre-diabetes.

25. **Avocados.** Avocados contain fats, but the good ones. So, never let yourself be deceived by its fat content because they are still good for you! Avocados are full of monounsaturated fat, the kind that helps slow the release of sugars into the bloodstream, prompting less insulin release.

26. **Chia Seed.** Chia seed stabilizes blood sugar, manages the effects of diabetes, improves insulin sensitivity, and aids symptoms related to metabolic syndrome. This includes imbalances in cholesterol, higher blood pressure,

and extreme rises in blood sugar levels after meals.

27.**Mangoes.** This fruit may taste so sweet but this delicious fruit may actually lower blood sugar according to research when taken in the right amounts.

28.**Olive oil.** Olive oil is usually used in beauty products, but surprisingly, this has good effects on our blood sugar level. Olive oil is rich in the same monounsaturated fat found in avocados, prevents not only belly fat accumulation, but also insulin resistance.

29.**Apple cider vinegar.** A spoonful of vinegar helps in lowering down your blood glucose level. According to studies, drinking a mixture of apple cider vinegar and water before eating has benefits. It helped increase sensitivity to insulin and reduced a spike in blood sugar after eating starchy food in those with pre-diabetes as well as those with type 2 diabetes.

30. **Eggs.** Clinical studies have found that overweight and obese people who were given two eggs a day for breakfast lost 65 percent more weight than those eating a similar breakfast without eggs. The researchers said eating eggs may control hunger by reducing the post-meal insulin response and control appetite by preventing large fluctuations in both glucose and insulin levels. Moreover, it has also been found that people who eat eggs for breakfast eat fewer calories for the entire day, as well as for the next 36 hours.

Chapter 6 - Muscle Up

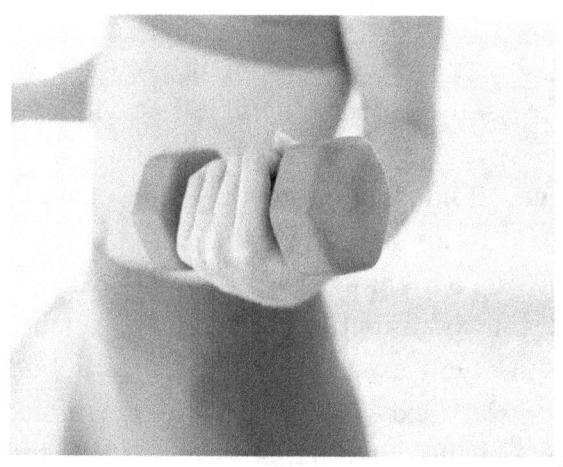

Muscles do wonderful things to your entire system. They hold your body together and help it move. Basically, to *muscle up* means that you have to stop being a couch potato – get up, move, and exercise! All forms of exercise do not only have positive effects on your physical aspect; it also has positive benefits on your wellbeing. It can actually provide a noticeable boost to your confidence and self-esteem. By setting and achieving your goals, you can help give yourself a greater sense of empowerment that will leave you feeling much happier and contented.

Also, exercising can help you relieve stress. It cannot be denied that when you are suffering from illnesses, you tend to over think, hence you become stressed. Stress can actually cause a number of health and mood problems. It can also diminish appetite and sleep quality. When you exercise, you force your body to exert excess energy and hormones. Exercising also helps you reduce your chances of developing tension headaches.

Here is a list of different exercises you can do to help you control your blood sugar level.

1. **Walking.** This is probably the most basic form of exercise. As they say, "walking is the best form of exercise". This is best for people who are just starting their road to fitness. Research says that you

only need 30 minutes of walking every day to maintain and improve good health. It helps you reduce the risk of coronary heart disease, risk of osteoporosis, breast cancer and colon cancer. Moreover, it helps patients improve blood pressure and blood sugar levels, improve blood lipid profile, maintain body weight and lower the risk of obesity, and it enhance mental wellbeing.

2. **Running.** Do not run think of running away from your problems, but literally run. Get that running shoes you kept for a long a time, because now is the best time to get back on track. Running is one of the most common exercises, not to mention that does not require you to pull out some cash from your wallet, unless you choose to do it in a sports complex. Running has a lot of benefits. Running regularly will help in improving

cardiovascular fitness, maintaining a healthy weight, in building strong bones. It strengthens your muscles which makes running incredibly effective at making you healthier in a number of ways. Whether you believe it or not, running actually increases your overall level of health. Studies have shown that running can raise your levels of good cholesterol while helping you increases lung function and use, at the same time. In fact, most doctors recommend running to those patients who are in the early stage of diabetes. In addition, running can also boost your immune system and lower your risk of developing blood clots.

3. **Strength Training.** This is the type of physical exercise which specializes in the use of resistance to induce muscular contraction that builds the strength, anaerobic endurance,

and size of skeletal muscles. This kind of training provides various functional benefits. It reduces the risk of developing diabetes and insulin needs, and lowers high blood pressure. Moreover, strength and weight training reduces stress and anxiety, and it decreases the chance of catching colds and illnesses. This kind of exercise also helps you develop a positive state of mind. You will begin to notice changes in your physical body, hence you will also develop a regular exercise routine in which your ability to handle stress effectively will improve. Furthermore, strength training allows you to sleep better; that is to fall asleep quicker and sleep deeper. Clinical studies have shown regular exercise to be one of the three best tools for effective stress management.

4. **Yoga.** While Yoga is oftentimes associated with meditation and spiritual activities, it is also a form of exercise that makes you sweat a lot without even noticing! It does not only increase focus and balance, it also improves your overall health. Yoga helps you lower your blood sugar level. Yoga lowers blood sugar and bad cholesterol and boosts good cholesterol. According to clinical studies, people with diabetes who do yoga are found to have relatively lower blood sugar compared to those who suffer from this illness who do not do yoga. Yoga lowers cortisol and adrenaline levels, encouraging weight loss, and improving sensitivity to the effects of insulin. Get your blood sugar levels down, and you decrease your risk of diabetic complications such as heart attack, kidney failure, and blindness. The other benefits of

yoga are: (1) improved flexibility, (2)increased blood flow, (3) protected spine, (4) build muscle strength, and (5) strengthened bones, and (4) Corrected posture.

5. **Dancing.** Yes, dancing helps you a lot and it does not require you to be a dancer. Dancing is one of the most enjoyable and entertaining type of exercise. It can be a way to stay fit for people of all ages, shapes and sizes. It improves the condition of your heart and lungs, muscle tone and strength. It also increases muscular endurance and motor fitness.

6. **Sports.** Engage yourself in sports—you may try basketball, volleyball, or baseball. Do not be afraid to join sports because just like other forms of exercise, this could help you control your blood sugar level.

Now that we have talked about ways of exercising, it is also important to know the proper techniques in performing those exercises.

1. First, you have to **seek advice from your physician** if your body is capable of doing such exercises— know the dos and don'ts first. So, it is important to have your check up before you start training.

2. When you do your exercises, remember to **always start by having a warm up**. It is always important to do warm up before you work out. A good warm up will gradually increase your heart rate, increase circulation to your muscles, tendons and ligaments, and will mentally prepare you for your workout. Also, it lessens the possibility of having muscle sore after your training.

3. **Do not overdo it.** Excessive physical activity can lead to injuries and could cause menstrual abnormalities to women. You may be exercising too much if your weight falls below normal or your muscles ache. In case of unbearable pain, seek help from your doctor.

4. **Drink of plenty water when exercising.** Drink at least two six-ounce glasses of water before, during and after working out. As you workout, you also release a lot of water from your body which could cause dehydration. Thus, it is important to drink water to rehydrate.

5. Lastly, **do not forget to always cool down** with stretching exercises. Just like doing warm up before starting your exercises, it is also important to end it through cool down. This will help prevent

injuries and unnecessary muscle sores.

Chapter 7 - Relax, Meditate, Sleep

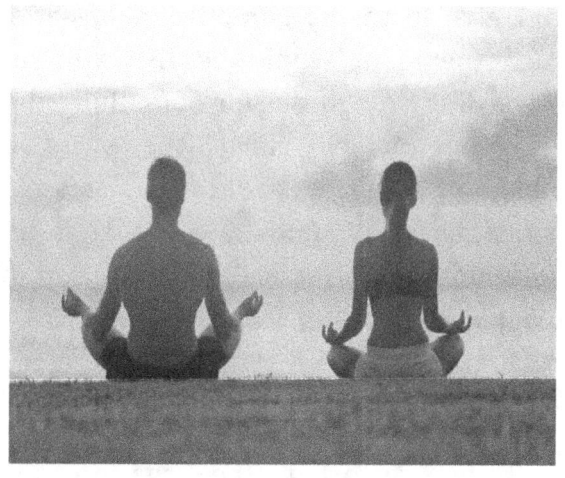

Aside from doing workout and exercise, your body also needs to relax because relaxation makes you feel less anxious or tense. Once you feel relaxed, it would be a lot easier for you to make adjustments, and become ready to face greater challenges.

Recognize it. Stress will be your number one enemy in facing this battle. Stress is evil, evil is stress. Stress brings with it a lot of evil in the world. It makes us do impulsive things, makes temptations irresistible, and worst of all stress could trigger a total relapse into addiction. If you give in to the compulsion of eating sugar again, it would be like you are rewarding your brain for something that is wrong which starts the cycle of addiction. Hence, avoid too stressful occasions at all times and if that is not possible then practice some relaxation techniques.

Knowing how to relax is vital for ensuring and maintaining a healthy wellbeing, as well as restoring the passion and happiness in your life.

1. **Recognize the stress.** You could be so stressed if all you think about is work, studies, career and all other things you are unsure of. It could be manifested through constant body tension, as well as neck aches, headaches, general soreness, and back aches. You are also often irritable, uneasy, hot-

tempered, and these could be the reason why you lose focus on completing various tasks. Trivial things set you off easily. However, not all stress is bad. There are times when we experience good stress, or what we call as eustress. It adds interest, excitement, thrill, and motivation to life, in the right balance.

2. **Take time to chill and relax.** When you recognize your stressors, it would be easy for you to accept the negative things impacting your life. Hence, it is important to have a place for relaxation amidst your business. First, you have to let go of that guilt. Sometimes, people find themselves guilty when they start to relax and try to at least escape work for a while. But, remember that hard work is giving your tasks the attention they deserve at the

time they deserve, not letting it bleed into all hours of your day!

3. **Practice breathing techniques.** Everything is so fast- paced right now so, do not even include your breathing to that. Slow down your breathing and actively concentrate on it. This is always the easiest way to self-calm, provided you remember to resort to it. You can do belly breathing. Just place your hands on your stomach and when you breathe in: you try to push away your hands, and when you breathe out you make your hands go towards you. Also, you may breathe in through your nose and out through your mouth. Do relax your muscles and nerves, inhale deeply as you count to five, hold your breath for five seconds, then exhale slowly, counting to five and repeat this ten times. Visualize the stress and tension leaving your body as you breathe out.

4. **Go for a ride.** You are probably preoccupied with a lot of things to do. However, you should never forget that you deserve a treat, you deserve a break. Hence, go for a ride. May it be through biking around your town or city, or long bus rides where a very beautiful destination awaits you. Travel. Explore. Live. And take time to appreciate the wonderful things that surround you!

5. **Try a massage.** Massage is a general term for pressing, rubbing and manipulating your skin, muscles, tendons and ligaments. Studies suggest that massage in an effective treatment for reducing stress, pain and muscle tension. This also helps in the flow and circulation of blood. Other benefits of massage are: reduces anxiety, headaches, and digestive disorders.

6. **Listen to a relaxing music.** Clinical studies have shown that music heals and it helps people with high blood sugar level have a more positive outlook in life. Music and rhythms are just as powerful as words of wisdom from of friends, families, and loved ones. It could move us to tears or makes us smile, and could stir up our minds, feelings and emotions. Studies suggest that music have positive effects on pain management. Music can help reduce both the sensation and distress of both chronic pain and postoperative pain. Furthermore, music has repulsive effects. It helps regulate the patients' blood flow and circulation. And music helps us relax by slow breathing and normal heartbeat, especially slow music. Have you noticed that when you attend parties, the music is too loud causing your heart to beat faster than normal? Same logic

happens when we listen to slow and classic music. It helps us have a normal heart beat.

7. **Practice positive thinking.** With all the negative things happening in your life, it is but necessary to fill your mind with good and happy thoughts. When you are optimistic, it does not mean that you are becoming too idealistic, and that you fantasize too much. Moreover, it is not about wishful or dreamer thinking; it is about making the most of the situations that you find yourself in and avoiding any tendency to add negative overlays.

8. **Practice meditation.** All thoughts and emotions should be removed from your body and mind by concentrating. Now, breathe. Meditation allows you to focus on your whole being, rather than just focus on one area of your body as any other relaxation technique

tends to do. It can take a while to master, but it is well worth the effort.

9. **Smile and laugh.** Laughter is the best medicine, as they say. This is guaranteed to help. Smiling and laughing releases endorphins, which fights stress, helps to you to relax and reminds you that life is more than just work. Although it feels strange at first, you have made it a point to smile more often.

10. **Surround yourself with positive people.** Spend time with those people who would bring out the best in you. Those kind of people **who radiate warmth and with whom you can truly connect.** Contact with positive-thinking and joyous people broadens your capacities enormously and helps you to feel more relaxed and happy.

11. **Have a long and good night sleep.** One of the factors that could trigger your wants of eating sweets and one of the things that make you more vulnerable to addiction is the lack of sleep. Sleep is necessary to keep your brain energized for the next day. Sleep restores and refreshes your body in myriad ways that cannot happen when you're awake. Do not be tempted to devalue the worth of sleep. When we sleep, our brain cells goes through the process of rewiring to integrate all our experiences and learning's of the day into memory. So in turn, when you sleep you start the creation of new memories and new habits which will make it easier for you to eat healthier and practice a better lifestyle. But never over sleep because it is not good for our health as well and make sure you have plenty of physical exercises as these will help in

reducing stress and creating a healthy tiredness that will in turn make you sleep tightly. You may also try yoga and swimming to improve your ways of sleeping.

Here are some other tips on how to improve your quality of sleep:

√Have a warm bath or shower before going to bed.

√Have an early dinner and avoid eating a heavy meal before sleeping.

√Drink plenty of water during the day.

√As much as possible, keep your bedroom cool and quiet.

√Choose to drink tea instead of coffee before going to bed.

Chapter 8 - Keep It Going

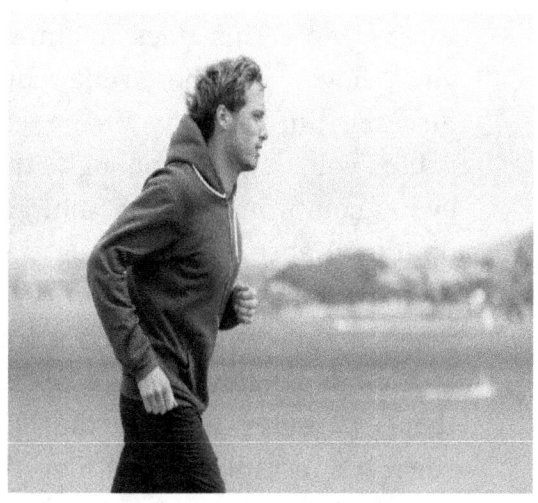

Most people have this tendency to do best when they are just starting, yet find it very difficult to maintain what they have started. If you want to really achieve change, then you have to turn your life 180 degrees, not in a blink of an eye, but through hard work and through time.

1. **Discipline.** Yes, discipline is very much important. Without it, you will not be able to move forward and totally change your bad habits

into good ones. When people offer you things you think may have bad effects on your health, learn how to say "no". This does not mean you have to be rude and disrespectful, it only means you value your health enough that even compromising is not an option. Hence, when you start saying "no" to temptation even when you do not want to, eventually you are going to believe that you really do not want the sugary substance. It is like the saying, "fake it 'til you make it".

2. **List down the reasons why sugar is bad for you and you have to memorize it.** Just like goal setting, you also have to list down all the reasons why sugar is not good for your health, in this way; it will be easier for you to make better choices. Deciding to change the course of our lives is not something we could easily do. It

takes time, and of course a lot of patience. There is always that moment of epiphany where you started looking the other way. Remember that moment, write it down, and remind yourself of that every single day.

3. **Seek help from really strict yet caring friends.** Going into this challenge of giving up sugar is not an easy thing to do; in fact it will seem almost impossible. There will be times, especially at the beginning, where it will almost be too difficult to continue. It will use up all your willpower and will ask for more. But you really do not have to go through it alone; you will need the help of friends or any form of social support. That's why you need to have strict friends who also truly care about you because they will help keep you in line, prevent you from picking up

that cupcake, and motivate you to keep going.

4. **Join or subscribe to health-related support groups, or communities.** When you are in this point of your life, you often feel alone and that no one understands what you are going through. But you may be surprised by how many people from around the world actually do. There are so many online sites with professional medical practitioners and bloggers who have had the same experience and are very much willing to share their knowledge on how you could control your blood sugar levels. People who share the same sentiments and experience with you will make you realize that you are not alone in your struggles and battle, and that there are people out there who suffer from diseases like you do yet they managed to be

happy and contented with their lives. The people you will encounter will help you mold a new perspective and inspire you to quit and leave bad habits behind and start a healthier you.

5. **Avoid and control a relapse.** Taking everything in moderation and maintaining the mindset of sugar as a reward rather than a necessity is the key to avoiding a major relapse. Not taking in sugar is very much impossible, since almost everything we consume have sugar even just a small amount. So it is really important to know your limitations.

6. **Reward yourself.** Liking sugar so much starts when the brain confuses but at the same time deceives itself into thinking that sugar is a necessity instead of a want. By this time it will be hard for you to resist consuming loads

of sugar. So, it is important to change your thinking that you need sugar. Instead, sugar should serve as a reinforcement and a reward for good behavior. Once you adapt a sugar-free regimen, you can reinforce your good behavior of sticking with it by giving yourself or having a friend give you a small treat. In psychology, this is referred to as the *token economy* where you have a set of conditions and a schedule when to eat something sweet. You can start slow with something like this: "I will eat ONE piece of chocolate candy if I get through a week without sugar". Then you can increase the challenge until you do not need them anymore.

7. **Keep yourself motivated; and do not stop until you get used to your new lifestyle.** If there's one thing you should regret about being a sugar dependent person, is

that it never goes away. This is something that you have to deal with and face for the rest of your life. Fortunately, you should believe that time heals all wounds, and that through time and you will be able to start anew. Later on, the impulses will be easier to handle and you will form new habits. But still, you should never let yourself forget what you have been through because it will inspire you even more. And most importantly, you should never stop motivating yourself to live a healthier life.

8. **Maturity.** One should be mature enough in dealing changes in his or her life. Also, you must be mature in choosing your life choices, and must always see the larger picture of the effects of your decisions rather than the short term effects.

9. **Stop saying tomorrow. Start now!** Now that you have read all

the ways, techniques, and methods of controlling your blood sugar level, you no longer have an excuse. Start applying any of them now. Test out the effectiveness of each one then try a combination of techniques and then mix it up a little when it gets boring.

CONCLUSION

Thank you again for downloading this book!

Having a high blood sugar level is just a problem with many, different solutions. At the end of the day, it is still you who is decisive. It is still you who has the freedom to make choices in life. But always keep in mind that your choices make and reveal you.

A lot of good things can happen to you and your family once you decide to take a 180 degrees turn from your previous lifestyle and habits. Life is one of the most wonderful gifts our God has given to us and do not waste it anyhow by indulging yourself into selfish doings. Having a high blood sugar level is just one of the struggle life has but that does not mean you always have to give up. To tell you honestly, the process of achieving health goal is not easy. It is never easy, but in the end, it will all be worth it. Every day is a constant battle between your "love" for your old lifestyle, and your love for yourself and your health. Life was never meant to be easy. It may throw balls at you; it may push you through your limits, and will attempt to break you down, but in the end, the difficulties you have experienced will make you a better person. Just always remember to put a good fight and always place your best foot forward!

Everything is just a matter of choice and a matter of having a good perspective. If you think your choices right now do not make you and your family feel secure, you better change your choices. Choose to live healthily because living that way ensures you a bright future.

Hopefully, everything that has been provided in this book will be instilled in your mind, and especially in your heart. I hope this will help you gain the confidence needed to start taking that first step: making a choice.

Also, I hope that this book has made you realize that it is still possible to change and that it is not yet too late to live a healthy life.

Every day, we are bombarded with so many choices. Thus, starting now, make the right choice and begin while you still can!

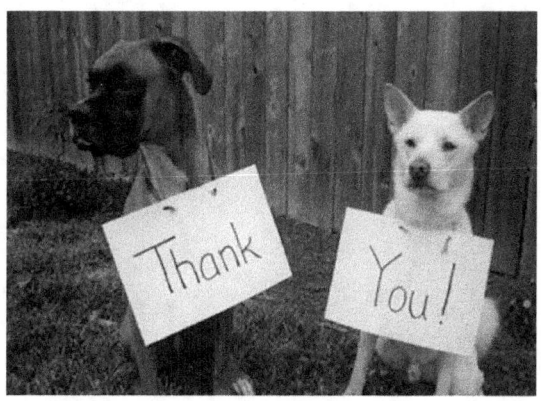

Finally, if you enjoyed this book, then I'd like to ask you for a favor, would you be kind enough to leave a review for this book on Amazon? It'd be greatly appreciated!

Click here to leave a review for this book on Amazon!